GOD IN PSYCHIATRY

The Mystery of Suffering and of Being Born Again

Thomas Hora, M.D.

The PAGL Foundation, Inc.

New York, NY

2013

The PAGL Foundation, Inc.

ISBN 0-913105-06-6
ISBN series 978-09131050-61
The PAGL Foundation, Inc.
New York, New York

CONTENT

INTRODUCTION	5
THEISTIC EXISTENTIALISM	9
HUMANISTIC PSYCHOLOGY	12
THE RIGHT MAN	13
CONCEPTS OF GOD	15
KNOWING THE UNIMAGINABLE	17
SPIRITUAL FACULTIES OF PERCEPTION	19
EXPANDING OUR MENTAL HORIZON	22
A BENEFICIAL PRESENCE	25
THE MYSTERY OF SUFFERING	26
ARE WE THINKING OUR OWN THOUGHTS?	28
TWO SOURCES OF THOUGHTS	30
PARENTAL FANTASIES	32
DEFINITIONS	33

INTRODUCTION

Thomas Hora, M.D., (1914-1995), was a psychiatrist with a passion for seeking spiritual understanding. His search led him beyond psychology to study philosophy, phenomenology, world religions and other existential and metaphysical teachings. The spiritual teachings of Jesus Christ became the cornerstone of his practice that he called Metapsychiatry.

Metapsychiatry offers a unique method of spiritual growth and understanding that manifests in healing of all kinds. It is not a religion. Dr. Hora's patients and students included followers of diverse religions, as well as non-religious individuals.

From 1983 to 1987 a group of his students* led by Jan Linthorst, D. Min., distilled the essence of this wisdom on twelve vital subjects and published them as a series of booklets, of which this is one. These, as well as books of Dr. Hora are available at www.Amazon.com. Audio recordings of classes with Dr. Hora are available through the PAGL Foundation at: www.pagl.org. PAGL is an acronym for Peace, Assurance, Gratitude, and Love. The presence of PAGL in consciousness, as taught in Metapsychiatry, is evidence of the existence of God and can be seen as a way by which to measure individual spiritual progress.

*Ann Linthorst, Joan Taylor, Joan Rubadeau and Gloria Spurgeons

Motto:

In the multitude of dreams and many words, there are also diverse vanities: but hear thou God

(Ecclesiastes 5:7).

THEISTIC EXISTENTIALISM

Recently, someone asked the following question: "Dr. Hora, you write and talk about existential theism as the basis of Metapsychiatry. It seems though, that wherever I turn in reading about existentialism, it does not seem to be in vogue to talk about God. And as for existentialism, it surfaced as a movement in the 1950's, but it was soon passed over, and now people are more interested in behaviorism or other philosophical approaches. Could you say something about the meaning of this?"

To be precise, we are not talking about existential theism but theistic existentialism. If we were talking about existential theism, we would be studying theology. If we talk about theistic existentialism, we are talking about a philosophy which takes into consideration the existence of God. The answer to the above question, however, is that there are more theistic existentialists among philosophers than meets the eye.

Existentialism is a widely misunderstood philosophical orientation and also much maligned. As for God, people are largely disillusioned with the concept. Various conventional religions have discredited the idea of God; therefore, philosophers who want to be accepted or listened to, prefer to present existentialism as a humanistic philosophy or as an atheistic philosophy or a crypto-theistic philosophy.

What is "crypto-theistic philosophy"? It is a philosophy where the issue of God is hidden. It is not mentioned openly. One of the most outstanding crypto-theistic philosophers was Heidegger, a former Catholic priest, who later became a philosopher and a rather brilliant one. What he did was to hide God under a cloud of obscure language. Once an interviewer asked him, "What is your position in regard to God?" In his customary fashion Heidegger said, "As for God, I am waiting for Him."

Interestingly enough, in many parts of the world, there is a certain degree of embarrassment about admitting interest in God. There are two existential philosophers who are forthright enough about their attitude towards God — the Roman Catholic philosopher, Gabriel Marcel and the Jewish philosopher, Martin Buber. As for Sartre, it is well known that he was openly and assertively atheistic. As far as psychiatry is concerned, God is almost totally absent. It seems unbecoming to a scientist to mention God because God is not subject to scientific experimentation. Consequently, in medicine and psychiatry, we hear very little about God.

Our culture in the United States is highly pragmatic and mostly humanistic in spite of the fact that our founding fathers were religious, God-fearing people. We tend to ignore God. We relegate Him to formal ceremonies on Sundays and holidays. God does not seem to be part of our everyday living.

In Metapsychiatry (which means "going beyond present-day psychiatry"), we study the relevancy of God-consciousness to mental health and healing processes, involving all aspects of life. We are endeavoring to put soul into psychiatry and breathe life into the "valley of dry bones." And, indeed, experience has proven that this way of seeking to understand man and his problems is very helpful.

A great deal of research has gone into the study of man. Man has been studied as a cadaver, as a machine, as a psychological organism, as a bio-chemical laboratory, and lately, man is being studied even as a molecular structure. All sorts of sophisticated and impressive research approaches have been devised for the study of man. Thus, we seem to know more and more about less and less. The scientific study of man over the years has proven itself quite frustrating. With all the miracles of modern science, we still live in fear of disease, decrepitude and above all, fear of treatment. The fact is that we still don't understand man. He remains a mystery.

The explanation of this, however, is simple. It is impossible to understand man by studying man. There is no such thing as man; there is only man in God, just as there is no leaf apart from a tree. If we want to understand a leaf, we must study the tree. To understand man, we must consider God, because God is the context in which man exists. There is no such thing as man apart from God. What happens to a leaf if we separate it from the tree? It ceases to be a leaf; it becomes trash. Thus, man can only be understood in the context of God, the creative Power, the Intelligence which sustains and constitutes his being. Therefore, Metapsychiatry studies man as a manifestation of divine existence.

Traditional psychiatry has mostly studied the

sicknesses of man. It is not unlike trying to understand a tree by studying the decaying processes of fallen leaves. Metapsychiatry proposes to study the life of man in the context of its life-giving source. Our primary interest is to come to understand healthy man. We are interested in knowing under what conditions man can be healthy. So we are not asking, What's wrong with man? but, What constitutes healthy man? It stands to reason that if we could understand the condition under which a healthy man can be found, this knowledge might prove to be extremely helpful and practical.

HUMANISTIC PSYCHOLOGY

Now the question is, in a humanistic and pragmatic culture as ours seems to be, is this idea acceptable? Not readily. Most people are interested in learning how to handle life. They are interested in managerial skills and how to operate. Few are interested in finding out what life is. Humanism is somewhat better than operationalism. Humanism says, "Man needs to be humanized. It is not enough to know how to handle people; we must invent certain values which will make man more amenable to the socializing process, so that he can live in communities with relative tolerance of his fellow man." While the operationalist dehumanizes man and turns him into an object of manipulation, the humanist civilizes man, but equally disregards the divine context, the creative matrix of existence. Humanism assumes that man can become a decent person through his own efforts and can get along with his fellow men just by wanting to.

Recently someone said, "I don't know what's the matter with me; I am trying to be generous and every morning in the office I volunteer to make coffee. Everybody comes to drink the coffee, but I have the feeling that people are just taking advantage of my generosity and disregarding me. The harder I try to be nice and generous, the less people appreciate it." This is an example of a humanistic endeavor to be generous and good. This man's idea of generosity was to be nice to people in the hope that they, in turn, would be nice to him and appreciate his helpfulness. But instead of that, he found that this kind of human generosity does not seem to work, since people just consider him a fool, or they see through his ulterior motive, namely, that humanistic generosity is just a public relations ploy.

In ancient China, there lived a sage called Chuang-tsu, who said, "If the wrong man does the right thing, then the right thing works the wrong way." Humanistic generosity creates the wrong man who is doing the right thing, but it works the wrong way. Therefore, social ethics are clearly not enough. It is not enough to be a "nice guy." The same Chuang-tzu reformulated his saying by putting it this way: "But if the right man happens to do the wrong thing, even the wrong thing may work the right way".

THE RIGHT MAN

Now the question is, What does it mean to be the "right man"? If we knew how to be the right man, then "all things would work together for good." (And we know that "all things work together for good to them that love God" (Romans 8:28). When it comes to generosity, what is the difference between the right and the wrong man? Someone said that the wrong man is trying to impress others, while the right man is trying to express God. That is beautiful and true, but it still describes man in behavioristic terms. Essentially, the difference is in the perspective.

The right man has an entirely different viewpoint on life and on himself than the wrong man. The wrong man's perspective on life is interpersonal, horizontal — self and others. The right man sees himself as an expression of divine Love-Intelligence, and his generosity is radically and qualitatively different.

Here, in a nutshell, we can see the principle of existential Metapsychiatry, which endeavors to help man become aware of himself as an expression, a manifestation of an existentially valid context in which he "lives and moves (and acts) and has his being" (Acts 17:28). Therefore, our work consists of helping people become "the right man." A "right man" cannot help but be a beneficial presence in the world, which is not synonymous with being a do-gooder. A do-gooder is the wrong man trying to do good. The right man is not a do-gooder; he is a "be-gooder." We are not learning how to do good, but how to be good, the good which we already are. Because if man is the image and likeness of God, a manifestation of divine Love-Intelligence, he cannot help but be good. His presence in the world is a blessing.

Thus, theistic existentialism can be fully appreciated in juxtaposition to pragmatism, operationalism, humanism, personalism, intellectualism, etc. We do not propose to change people; we just help them realize the perfection which underlies their essential being. "Be ye therefore perfect, even as your Father which is in heaven is perfect" (Matthew 5:48).

CONCEPTS OF GOD

Since Metapsychiatry is based on the metaphysical definition of man within the context of God, it is naturally important to have a very clear and existentially valid concept of God. There are many concepts of God, and they are mostly religious concepts. In the Old Testament, God appears to be first a frightful judge, a warlord and a legalistic authority. Later on, He is gradually becoming more benevolent and less punitive until, with the advent of Jesus, he becomes a loving Father. In fact, we can view the Bible as a record of man's evolving concept of God.

The more primitive the mentality of man is, the more frightful, intimidating and even monstrous is his god, and vice versa. But Jesus speaks of God as a loving Father. Here we can already breathe a little easier, but still there is the problem of anthropomorphism. We could ask, What prompted Jesus to speak of God as a Father and thus give rise to male supremacist fantasies and reinforce the tendency towards anthropomorphism? We can theorize that the reason for this may have been the fact that Jesus was talking to primitive people who were not sufficiently evolved to conceive of infinity or the possibility of an intelligence and power governing the universe and having no form.

It took many centuries for human consciousness to develop the capacity for abstract thinking and to conceive of a power and of an intelligence which is infinite, because infinity cannot be imagined. The moment we try to imagine something, it must assume a form. The non-dimensional cannot be imagined. Therefore, it is very difficult, even today, for the average religious individual to conceive of God as infinite Presence, infinite Power, an infinite Intelligence.

There was one man who went beyond Jesus in his definition of God. It was John, who defined God as Love — not someone who loves, but simply Love. Thus, he is the first one to define God as a quality. Qualities do not have form. Here we already reach an evolutionary stage where human consciousness is able to speak of God without ascribing it form.

It is interesting to remind ourselves that among the ten commandments in the Old Testament, we find it prohibited to make "graven images" of God. "Graven images" refers to a mental process based on the power of imagination. In fact, it is a prohibition against the attempt to visualize God in some finite form. It is noteworthy that this commandment appears at a time when human consciousness was not yet ready to behold the nondimensional. In order for something to be thought, it had to have form. Abstract thinking was not a common ability. Undoubtedly, there were unique individuals in ancient Egypt and in the Orient who were able to conceive of the nondimensional and the infinite, but this was not true of the average human being.

In order to understand God in an existentially valid way — and this is crucial — it is necessary to reach a level of mental development where one is comfortable with the idea of the nondimensional. We must come to know the unimaginable God, because that which can be imagined is purely imaginary, and we are not dealing with imaginary things; we seek to apprehend Reality.

KNOWING THE UNIMAGINABLE

To understand man in the context of God, it is important to understand that God is unimaginable Reality; we have to be capable of knowing that which cannot be imagined. This may appear somewhat frightening, but actually it is not too difficult. In Metapsychiatry we speak of God as Love-Intelligence. Love-Intelligence is a cosmic force constituting ultimate Reality. It cannot be given a form; it is impossible. This Love-Intelligence is the creative power from which everything real emanates. And man, as the image and likeness of God, is likewise unimaginable. The man that can be imagined is not man but a phenomenon, namely an appearance. The famous Zen Master, Suzuki, used to startle his students with the mind-boggling statement, "Form is formlessness and formlessness is form."

Form as phenomenon is misleading and distracting and thus interfering with true perception. Jesus warned us, "Judge not according to the appearance, but judge righteous judgment" (John 7:24), which means if we judge man by his appearance, then we shall arrive at false conclusions about him, and this will give rise to many schools of psychotherapy. But if we judge righteous judgment, then there will be only one school of psychotherapy, because then we will know the truth of what man really is and the truth will make us free from errors.

Thus, in order to have a solid, existentially valid foundation for a school of psychotherapy or spiritual guidance, we must know man as he really is, namely in the context of God, for there is no such thing as a man apart from God. It is impossible to arrive at any valid understanding of man when he is studied out of context.

Recently, I asked an artist who was having some problems, whether he could paint a picture without a background. He said, "Of course, it is very simple. I just take an empty canvas and paint the foreground and leave out the background." He thought that if he did not paint the background, there was no background. But, of course, the empty canvas would be the background. It is impossible for anything to exist in the world in and of itself. It is impossible for man to exist without his creative background. And the creative background of man is infinite Love-Intelligence. And the background determines the foreground, always. The foreground has no power over the background.

Man, in the context of God, is revealed to be a manifestation of Love-Intelligence. God can also be spoken of as cosmic Consciousness. The quality of this infinite Love-Intelligence is consciousness and life itself. Cosmic Consciousness determines its infinite manifestations. Therefore, man is equipped with the capacity to be conscious. So, infinite cosmic Consciousness, which is the background, determines the foreground of an infinite variety of individualized consciousnesses. Man is a conscious expression of infinite Love-Intelligence. This is seeing man in the context of God.

SPIRITUAL FACULTIES OF PERCEPTION

The question may be asked, How can we see that which has no form and cannot be imagined? There is more to man than meets the eye. We all have the faculty to discern spiritual qualities in the world. We can see honesty; we can see integrity; we can see beauty; we can see love; we can see goodness; we can see joy; we can see peace; we can see harmony; we can see intelligence; and so forth. None of these things has any form; none of these things can be imagined; none of these things is tangible, and yet they can be seen. What is the organ that sees these invisible things? Some people call it the soul, spirit, or consciousness. Man is a spiritual being endowed with spiritual faculties of perception.

Recently, I worked with a young woman who was blind from childhood on, and I told her, "You can really think of yourself as a sighted individual because Reality is available to you to perceive. In fact, you are able to see Reality because you are just as able to discern the spiritual attributes which comprise Reality as anyone else. Your spiritual faculties of perception are unimpaired." This was of great comfort to her. At once she felt herself closer to the rest of humanity and to God. She realized that all the essential elements of Reality are available to her to be "seen."

Our spiritual faculties of perception constitute the real essence of the good life. Whatever is good in life, whatever is "happyfying," whatever is comforting, whatever is healing, whatever matters in life is the awareness of these spiritual attributes of Reality. There is no human being who is not spiritual, but the vast majority of people are so involved with experiential living that they are distracted from the awareness of the spiritual dimension.

There is a radical difference between what is mediated through the senses and has form, is imaginable and can be experienced, and that which is nondimensional, unimaginable, and cannot be experienced, but can be realized and spiritually discerned. It is universal Love-Intelligence, man's true dwelling place. The apostle Paul said, "While we look not at the things which are seen, but at the things which are not seen; for the things which are seen are temporal; but the things which are not seen are eternal" (II Corinthians 4:18).

The universal tendency and desire to "experience" life is a great distraction which prevents us from using our spiritual faculties of perception. When a metapsychiatrically oriented therapist sits down with a patient, he will not focus his attention on whether the patient is male or female, well-dressed or poorly dressed, educated or uneducated, tall or short, heavy or slim, etc. His focus will be on the reality of the individual, and his concern will be to help him wake up his faculties of spiritual discernment and discover himself in the right context. "Awake thou that sleepest, and arise from the dead, and Christ shall give thee light" (Ephesians 5:14).

So, the therapist views the patient in the context of absolute Reality and that helps him see himself in that context. When that realization is awakened in any one of us, everything becomes transformed and healed.

In Metapsychiatry, diseases are understood to be signs of misdirected modes of being-in-the-world. What we are helping people to be healed of, are their modes of being-in-the-world, regardless of diagnostic labels. Misdirected modes of being-in-the-world can be recognized, regretted, and reformed, and thus replaced by valid modes of being-in-the-world. These validate themselves through healings. Of course, no one can be healed against his will, and it would be arrogant and intrusive of a therapist to try to do so. The desire to be healed arises under two conditions: suffering and wisdom. Without these factors there is no motivation for healing, and the therapist has no right to attempt it.

In Metapsychiatry, we see man in a larger context. In conventional psychological thinking, man is seen as an autonomous unit, acting from his own mind and being affected by intrapsychic processes motivating him from the unconscious.

When we look at man as a psycho-physiological organism, then we see that indeed, there is such a thing as the unconscious. We do not see any place where the so-called unconscious could be located, but we are aware of the fact that there are many things we are not conscious of and there are things we are semi-conscious of, or more or less conscious of. Psychology would say, "What you don't know can hurt you." Thus, we say there is no unconscious, but there is unconsciousness. In Metapsychiatry, however, this is a trivial issue, because the moment we see man in a wider context — in the context of God — then this issue disappears and what we have is God, infinite cosmic Mind, completely determining man. "I and my Father are one" (John 10:3). "I am in the Father, and the Father in me" (John 14:11).

EXPANDING OUR MENTAL HORIZON

Many things which seem to be important in a narrower context, completely disappear when the mental horizon is expanded to a wider context. To illustrate, in Newtonian physics, cause and effect relationships are a matter of fact, and in our everyday lives everyone knows that there is cause and effect. However, when we expand our mental horizon, we discover that there is really no such thing as cause and effect relationship. In Metapsychiatry, we seek to expand our mental horizon into the maximum possible dimension, namely, that of infinite Mind.

Let us consider, for instance an object which we let drop to the ground. If we ask, Why did the object fall down? we would be, in fact, asking what caused it to fall down. The answer is, the object dropped because it was let go of.

This seems like common sense cause and effect reasoning — and judging by appearances. This is an example of conventional reasoning. We always ask, Why do certain things happen? Why does someone have a headache? Why does someone fight with his employer? Why are we afraid of the dark?

In Metapsychiatry we understand that there is no such thing as cause and effect relationship. Therefore, we ask a different question: What is the meaning of what seems to be? So, if we ask, What is the meaning of an object dropping to the ground? we receive an answer saying, This phenomenon reveals the existence of an invisible force called gravitation. Asking the meaning is asking, What does it indicate, that objects tend to fall to the ground? We immediately recognize that at this moment our mental horizon has become much broader than it was previously, when reasoning from the standpoint of cause and effect. The cause and effect dimension of reasoning is narrow-minded; it is only applicable within certain circumscribed, limited perspectives on life. Therefore, it is very important to know what questions to ask.

Metapsychiatry has isolated six questions which have been designated as "futile" questions. These questions are universally asked in all schools of psychotherapy. As a result of these six futile questions, our perspective on life and reality remains limited. They keep us from expanding our mental horizon. These questions are as follows: What's wrong? How do you feel? Why? Who is to blame? What should I do? How should I do it? We have taken these questions for granted, and it is time now to question their validity. We are born ignorant and we are educated to become increasingly so.

Just as cause and effect reasoning disappears in the context of cosmic Consciousness, so the issue of conscious and unconscious thinking also fades away, and many other things tend to disappear when the mental horizon becomes wide enough.

We may now ask, If these six questions which are the foundation of conventional reasoning are eliminated, what is there left? How are we going to function in psychotherapy and in life? Is it possible to live and function intelligently without these common sense questions? Is it practical? Yes, it is. In Metapsychiatry we found two very useful intelligent questions. These are: What is the meaning of what seems to be? And, What is what really is?

These two questions underlie and make possible the hermeneutic process of clarification which is the basic method of metapsychiatric therapy. To illustrate, a man comes seeking help for a marital problem. His marriage had deteriorated into a continuous state of discord. He was hoping that the psychiatrist would find a way of straightening out his wife and making her do what he wanted her to do. In talking to this man, who happened to be a salesman and a hockey player, he revealed a certain mode of being-in-the-world which could be best described as a "steam roller." It was pointed out to him that while he professed to be seeking guidance, he never gave the doctor a chance to get a word in edgewise, and that he continuously endeavored to instruct the doctor on how he should "handle" his wife. After a while, it was pointed out to him that he was not really a hockey player and not even a salesman because God never created such people. He happened to be a victim of miseducation concerning his own true nature, which is that of a man who expresses peace, assurance, gratitude, love, and intelligence. At first, he found this unbelievable, but slowly he began to see that his marital discord revealed his misdirected mode of being-in-the-world and that this could be healed just as soon as he discovered the truth of his own being.

Many who read this may be tempted to redefine what they are reading in terms of what they already know. Someone may say, "But this is nothing new; it is no different from what others do. It is just a different vocabulary and attitude." What follows is an example of this tendency to put "new wine into old bottles".

A BENEFICIAL PRESENCE

In Metapsychiatry mental health is defined as "being a beneficial presence in the world." Whenever this definition is presented to an audience, shortly thereafter someone will invariably "correct" or redefine it by speaking of a "beneficent person." When we inquire as to the meaning of this phenomenon, it is revealed to us that the concept of "beneficent person" is more in keeping with conventional thinking, which is operational and personalistic. Conventional psychological thinking views man as a self-existent personality, acting autonomously in the world, independent of God. But Metapsychiatry says, "Let us expand our mental horizon and behold man in the context of God, infinite Love-Intelligence."

A beneficial presence is not an operator, neither does he assume attitudes. We cannot make ourselves into beneficial presences. It is a quality of being, arrived at through a liberated consciousness. What is our consciousness to be liberated from? We need to be liberated from the narrow confines of conventional thinking. The bars of our prison window are built of the six futile questions.

Someone once remarked, "The worst thing that ever happened to me was when I was 18 years old and read Dale Carnegie's book. How to Win Friends and Influence People. I memorized his principles and began to use them very successfully. But the total operationalism of this approach led to a tremendous sense of isolation, because I could see I was using a technique on my friends. I was a practicing beneficent person. That was a real trap where social success was existential failure."

Thus, seeing life in a narrow context — cause and effect thinking, operationalism, the six futile questions — can lead to much suffering.

THE MYSTERY OF SUFFERING

What is suffering? In general, we can say that suffering is an unpleasant experience; it can be physical, emotional, mental, social, economic, personal, interpersonal, conscious, unconscious, acute, chronic, mild or severe. We can distinguish seven elements in suffering: (1) the cause of suffering (2) the meaning of suffering (3) the purpose of suffering (4) the sources of suffering (5) the essence of suffering (6) the remedy for suffering (7) the common denominator of all suffering.

1. The cause of suffering: The most primitive reaction to suffering is to ask, Why? or What is the cause of our suffering? This is very simplistic. We can usually find something to explain our suffering and someone to blame for it. This may make us feel somewhat better, but it really doesn't solve our problem. Cause and effect reasoning is inadequate for real understanding of the experience.

2. The meaning of suffering: In Metapsychiatry, we go beyond cause and effect reasoning and seek to understand the meaning of our experience. We have discovered that experiences are thoughts perceived organismically. Therefore, we approach every problem with the question, What is the meaning of this phenomenon? or What is the meaning of what seems to be?

3. The purpose of suffering: Having discovered that all suffering is meaningful, it is understandable that it also has a purpose. The purpose of suffering is to teach us something we must come to know of Reality and how to live in greater harmony with it. One of the metapsychiatric principles states: "Problems are lessons designed for our edification."

4. The sources of suffering: The sources of suffering are the "five gates of hell" (sensualism, emotionalism, intellectualism, materialism, and personism); the "four horsemen" (envy, jealousy, rivalry and malice); selfishness and unselfishness; wanting and not wanting; what should be and what shouldn't be; judging and not judging, self-confirmatory ideation.

5. The essence of suffering: The essence of suffering can be found in the word "agony." The metapsychiatric analysis of this word reveals that it means "lack of knowing." "A" comes from "alfa privativum," indicating "lack, absence or being without" something; the word "gony" in Latin is derived from "cognocere," which means "to know." We are all familiar with the term "agnostic," meaning "claiming ignorance of God." So, the essence of human suffering is the agony of unenlightened living.

6. The remedy for suffering: The remedy for agony or suffering is theogony, which means the true knowledge or understanding of God. The story of Job is very instructive in this regard. Job, who was a very decent man, a religious

Jew, suffered greatly. He was afflicted with boils and a variety of personal tragedies and couldn't understand why he should have to suffer so much. He kept crying out to God, "Show me my guilt," but there was no answer to this question; neither was there any acceptable comforting explanation from his well-meaning friends. At last he reached a point where he could say, "I have known Thee by the hearing of the ear, but now mine eye seeth Thee." In other words, his agonies yielded to the emergence of theogony.

7. The common denominator of all suffering: in Metapsychiatry it is called self-confirmatory ideation. This term is somewhat analogous to the theological concept of original sin; however, we do not ascribe to it a notion of culpability. It is simply a universal tendency of unenlightened man to be here for himself and to be mentally preoccupied with self-preservation and self-promotion, thus losing sight of his existential context, which is God.

In an existential context, suffering can be useful if it leads to a transformation which Jesus has described as being born again.

ARE WE THINKING OUR OWN THOUGHTS?

A beautiful young woman said, "I want to be liked, but when I succeed in getting people to like me, I feel extremely uncomfortable. I don't know how to lose interest in wanting to be liked. It seems so important, and yet it makes me feel very uneasy."

It is generally believed that it is normal to want to be liked, yet it can be a problem. How can that which is "normal" be problematic? The young lady was asked who was making her do the things which she did in order to be liked. She answered, "My thoughts." Then she was asked, "How do you know that those are your thoughts?" She said, "Because I am thinking them. It seems that being liked is something that I want. And yet it is a problem because part of me resents it."

Now, this example makes us ask, Are we thinking our own thoughts? It certainly seems so. But is it so? Is man a producer of thoughts? Are there any thoughts at all that are strictly our own? And how could we tell the difference?

Suppose the above-mentioned young woman had some less conventional thoughts; for example, suppose she were to think, "I want to be shorter than I am." She could possibly be driven by such thoughts to inflict injury on herself and seek surgery, or an accident or some disease to fulfill the demands of those thoughts. And she would still have the conviction that she was acting and bringing certain experiences into her life in accordance with her own thoughts. This brings to mind performances by hypnotists who give their subjects certain posthypnotic suggestions and simultaneously command them to believe that it is their own will they are acting upon. Now, such a subject cannot be freed of his post-hypnotic trance until he is helped to become aware of the fact that the suggested thoughts controlling him were not really his thoughts.

Similarly, one cannot be liberated from one's problems

until there is an awareness of the meaning and origin of the thoughts which exert their influence on an individual. If we realize that we are just living out someone else's fantasies, suggestions, personal values and wants, then one can turn away from them and wake up. It is, therefore, of great importance to ask, Are these my thoughts?

TWO SOURCES OF THOUGHTS

Metapsychiatry claims that man is not capable of producing his own thoughts. If this is true, then all our thoughts have come to us from somewhere else. Therefore, we are living in a state of hypnotism. We are living in a dream and dreaming dreams which have been suggested to us either overtly or covertly. It has been observed that Freudian patients tend to have Freudian dreams, Jungian patients Jungian dreams, etc.

The medieval physician, Paracelsus, observed that nothing can be in human consciousness except what enters through the five senses: "Nihil est in intellectu quod primum non fuerit in sensu." Of course, he was unaware of subliminal and extrasensory elements of communication. Furthermore, he conveniently ignored the possibility of God, or the divine Mind, as a source of creative ideas reaching human consciousness through inspiration. But these are still not our thoughts; they belong to God.

Therefore, in Metapsychiatry, we understand that thoughts have two sources. Invalid thoughts come from the "sea of mental garbage," where ignorant humans live and move and have their being, while valid thoughts come from the "ocean of Love-Intelligence," where enlightened man dwells. "Because thou hast made the Lord, which is my refuge, even the most High, thy habitation; there shall no evil befall thee, neither shall any plague come nigh to thy dwelling" (Psalms 91:10,11).

In Metapsychiatry, we learn to distinguish between existentially valid and invalid thoughts and thereby can safeguard our consciousness from pollutants. We are stewards of our consciousness and can preserve its purity. We cease to be victims of parental fantasies and human hypnotism. "Awake thou that sleepest, and arise from the dead, and Christ shall give thee light" (Ephesians 5:14). In this light we can see clearly that only God's thoughts constitute our true being. This realization is absolutely necessary in order for healings to take place.

A sophisticated psychiatrist could say all this is religious nonsense, encouraging people to become paranoid and hear their thoughts coming to them from an alien source in the form of hallucinations. Indeed, it is true that there are mentally disturbed people who are clearly aware that their thoughts are not their own, and they feel tormented and victimized by these hallucinations. But attempting to convince them that they are hearing their "own thoughts" has been utterly futile as a therapeutic approach. It seems much more helpful to invite them to learn to discriminate between valid ideas and invalid ideas, whatever their source and mode of entrance into awareness. As for hallucinations, we can understand that they are phenomena of the hypnotic trance, which can be deeper or shallower at different times, just like sleep. In sleep we all hallucinate. We call it dreaming.

PARENTAL FANTASIES

Normal, unenlightened life is a state of dreaming. Parental fantasies are communicated to the children either overtly or subliminally, verbally or nonverbally, with or without conscious intent. For instance, a child may come home from school with a diagnosis of dyslexia. From that moment on, she ceases to be a daughter to her highly educated parents. She becomes a clinical case to be studied anxiously and therapeutized at every turn. The result is catastrophic because the child becomes increasingly self-conscious and clumsy, full of rage and despair. From here on, her life is a dream of inadequacy and failure. "The fathers have eaten a sour grape, and the children's teeth are set on edge" (Jeremiah 31:29). Of course, the intentions are good, both in the parents and in the school system; however, ignorance and miseducation lead to suffering and even tragic consequences. Some children get programmed for disaster and some for success, some for poverty and some for riches, but no one is going to be happy or healthy as long as he lives the fantasies of his parents. That's what Jesus meant when he said to the 70-year-old Nicodemus, "Verily, verily, I say unto thee; except a man be born again, he cannot see the kingdom of God" (John 3:3). "I am come to set a man at variance against his father, and the daughter against her mother, and the daughter-in-law against her mother-in-law" (Matthew 10:2). "That which is born of the flesh is flesh; and that which is born of the Spirit is spirit" (John 3:6).

It has been clear since ancient times that the human experience is, by and large, unsatisfactory, self-contradictory and rather incomprehensible. "Man that is born of woman is of few days, and full of trouble" (Job 14:1). This realization has led to many philosophies and efforts to find ways of making sense out of life, and perchance to improve man's lot through some form of transformation. As a result we have a whole array of religious, philosophical and psychological systems which are recommended or believed in: reincarnation; transmigration of the soul; being born again; transfiguration; redemption; salvation; resurrection; curing, healing, conversion, etc.

DEFINITIONS

To bring some clarity into this profusion of ideas, we shall here attempt to define as many of these as would be helpful for our purposes. Looking at it from a metapsychiatric point of view, we can say the following:

1. Reincarnation is the materially human counterpart of being born again. It is a change from flesh to flesh. Every time we change our mode of self-confirmatory behavior, we are reincarnating ourselves into another material form. The most drastic instances of reincarnation today are cosmetic surgery and transsexualism.

2. Transmigration of the soul is a shift from one form of animality to another within the character structure of a primitive, individual consciousness. For instance, when someone who has lived as a "pussycat" deciles to become a "tiger."

3. Being reborn of the Spirit is synonymous with enlightenment. It entails realizing the true essence and substance of life in its individual manifestations. When Buddha was reborn of the Spirit he said, "I have now escaped the necessity of reincarnations forever." We understand this to mean that enlightened man loses the universal human urge for self-confirmatory ideation.

4. A cure is an attempt to repair a defective aspect of the human body or mind.

5. Healing is an endeavor to restore an individual to wholeness in terms of his mode of being-in-the-world.

6. Redemption is an endeavor to re-establish an individual's sense of self-worth.

7. Salvation is an endeavor to rescue an individual from a morally misdirected mode of being-in-the-world.

8. Transfiguration is the discernment of the fact that man is not the material form he seems to be.

9. Conversion is a changed perception of reality or certain aspects of reality. We can distinguish five forms of conversion:

(a) Sensory conversion occurs when an individual commits himself totally to a life of pleasure-seeking.

(b) Emotional conversion occurs when an individual becomes sentimental about, say, religion.

(c) Ideological conversion occurs when an individual discovers a different philosophy, theology or political doctrine than what he was previously attached to.

(d) Cognitive conversion occurs when someone, say an artist, begins to see some new aspects of reality and changes his way of expressing himself in his work.

(e) Spiritual conversion occurs when someone awakens to the reality of God as manifesting itself in spiritual values, qualities and ideas.

It is interesting to note that in most forms of conversion, individuals will say, "I have changed; I am not what I was before." However, in the case of spiritual conversion, the individual will say, "I am what I always was and always will be. I am what I am. I am a place where God's presence reveals itself as Love-Intelligence."

We see, then, that in contrast to Oriental religions, Jesus did not speak of reincarnation and transmigration of the soul. He demonstrated spiritual transformation on the mount of transfiguration and pointed to the absolute necessity of spiritual enlightenment as the ultimate answer to the human condition. "Marvel not that I said unto thee, ye must be born again" (John 3:7).

Metapsychiatry says, "Enlightened man is a "beneficial presence" in the world; he glows in the transcendental light of infinite Love-Intelligence."

This booklet is one of a series of twelve essays by Thomas Hora, M.D.

Healing Through Spiritual Understanding
A Hierarchy of Values
Forgiveness
The Soundless Music of Life
Can Meditation be Done?
Compassion
Marriage and Family Life
God in Psychiatry
What Does God Want?
Self-Transcendence
Right Usefulness
Commentaries on Scripture

Other books by Thomas Hora, M.D.

Encounters with Wisdom (Multi-Volume Set)
One Mind
Beyond the Dream
Dialogues in Metapsychiatry
Existential Metapsychiatry
In Quest of Wholeness

For more information about Metapsychiatry visit:
www.PAGL.org
or contact
The PAGL Bookstore
P.O. Box 4001
Old Lyme, CT 06371

Made in the USA
Monee, IL
04 November 2026

67383335R00022